A Guide to Overcoming Autoimmune Disease

Preventing and reversing chronic symptoms with nutritious foods

Brenda F. Dozier

Gratitude

Dear Reader,

It is with great gratitude that I extend my sincere thanks to you for deciding to start on this transformative path with "A Guide to Overcoming Autoimmune Disease: Preventing and Reversing Chronic Symptoms with Nutritious Foods." Your decision to explore these pages demonstrates a commitment to health, empowerment, and the pursuit of well-being.

This book is the outcome of a profound enthusiasm for holistic health and a desire to share knowledge that might positively benefit lives afflicted by autoimmune diseases. Your support and involvement with this content not only validate this aim but also contribute to a greater community of persons seeking strength and healing.

I am grateful for the opportunity to accompany you on this path toward greater health. Your drive to explore the nexus of nutrition, lifestyle, and autoimmune wellness is encouraging. Together, we can nurture resilience, accept optimism, and negotiate the intricacies of autoimmune problems with educated choices and transformative practices.

As you look into each chapter of this guide, may you find practical ideas, concrete tactics, and empowering viewpoints that resonate with your particular health path. Let us celebrate each step forward, no matter how tiny, and picture a future full of vigor, resilience, and joy.

Thank you once again for your trust and commitment to your health and well-being. I am happy to be a part of your support system and advocate for your journey toward conquering autoimmune difficulties with the power of healthy meals and holistic treatments.

With deep appreciation,

[Brenda *F. Dozier*].

Table of Contents

Introduction

Welcome to "A Guide to Overcoming Autoimmune Disease: Preventing and Reversing Chronic Symptoms with Nutritious Foods," which is a comprehensive resource on the subject. Autoimmune diseases are among the most challenging difficulties that have ever been encountered in the wide panorama of human health. These illnesses, which manifest themselves when the immune system of the body erroneously attacks its own tissues, are experienced by millions of people all over the world. They are characterized by a wide range of symptoms and complications that can have a substantial influence on the quality of life.

Imagine that your body is a perfectly tuned instrument, with each component functioning in harmony to keep your body in a state of perfect equilibrium and vitality. Imagining this balance being thrown off by the dissonance of autoimmune dysfunction, in which the body's defenses turn inward and launch an assault on its own cells and tissues, is a significant step toward understanding the situation. What is the end result? This condition is characterized by a chain reaction of inflammatory responses, chronic pain, exhaustion, and a wide variety of other incapacitating symptoms that can leave sufferers feeling helpless and overwhelmed.

There is, however, optimism in spite of the unpredictability and difficulties that are associated with autoimmune disorders. In the process of modifying immune function and alleviating the symptoms of autoimmune disorders, nutrition appears to play a vital role, according to the findings of recent research and clinical data. In fact, the foods that we eat have the ability to affect the expression of genes, control inflammation, and promote overall health and well-being.

This guide is your path to reclaiming control over your health and embarking on a journey toward recovery and vitality. Through the lens of nutrition and lifestyle interventions, we will discover the relationship between diet and autoimmune disease, finding the ways in which nutrient-rich foods can serve as effective allies in the fight against chronic illness.

Before we go into the practical solutions and insights presented within this chapter, let us first take a moment to grasp the nature of autoimmune disorders and the enormous impact they have on individuals and communities globally. By obtaining a deeper understanding of the mechanisms causing autoimmune dysfunction, we may better grasp the need to take a holistic approach to healing—one that treats the basic causes of illness while nourishing the body, mind, and soul.

Throughout this guide, we will rely upon the latest scientific research, clinical expertise, and real-life experiences to give you concrete counsel and practical solutions for managing and overcoming autoimmune diseases. Whether you are confronting the obstacles of a newly diagnosed ailment or seeking to enhance your health and well-being, this book is designed to empower you with the knowledge and tools needed to go on your road toward healing.

let's remember that healing is not a destination but a constant process—a journey of self-discovery, resilience, and progress. With dedication, perseverance, and the appropriate tools at your disposal, you have the capacity to rewrite the story of your health and hold a future full of energy, joy, and opportunity. So, without further ado, let's begin the incredible healing power of nutritious meals in the context of autoimmune disease.

Brief Explanation of Autoimmune Disease

Autoimmune diseases are a set of conditions characterized by the body's immune system mistakenly attacking its own tissues and organs. Normally, the immune system serves as the body's defensive mechanism, protecting against outside invaders such as bacteria, viruses, and other pathogens.

However, individuals with autoimmune illnesses, this defense system becomes dysregulated, leading to the generation of autoantibodies that target healthy cells and tissues.

Definition and Prevalence

Autoimmune disorders cover a vast array of conditions, each with its own distinct set of symptoms, triggers, and repercussions. While the specific origin of autoimmune illnesses remains unclear, experts believe that a combination of genetic predisposition, environmental factors, and dysregulated immune responses contribute to their development.

The prevalence of autoimmune disorders is on the rise, with millions of persons globally impacted by these conditions. According to the American Autoimmune Related Illnesses Association (AARDA), there are over 100 recognized autoimmune illnesses, impacting nearly 50 million Americans alone. Furthermore, autoimmune illnesses disproportionately affect women, with females accounting for around 75% of diagnosed cases.

Common Types and Their Symptoms

Autoimmune illnesses show in a wide variety of forms, each with its own unique set of symptoms and clinical manifestations. Some of the most prevalent autoimmune disorders include rheumatoid arthritis, lupus, multiple sclerosis, psoriasis, celiac disease, Type 1 diabetes, and Hashimoto's thyroiditis, among others.

Common Autoimmune Conditions

1. Rheumatoid Arthritis (RA): RA is a chronic inflammatory illness that mostly affects the joints, producing pain, swelling, stiffness, and limited mobility. Over time, RA can lead to joint degeneration and deformity, greatly reducing an individual's quality of life.

2. Lupus (Systemic Lupus Erythematosus): Lupus is a systemic autoimmune illness that can affect various organs and tissues, including the skin, joints, kidneys, heart, lungs, and brain. Common symptoms of lupus include weariness, joint discomfort, skin rashes, fever, and organ inflammation.

3. Multiple Sclerosis (MS): MS is a neurological autoimmune disease marked by damage to the protective myelin layer protecting nerve fibers in the brain and spinal cord. This injury affects nerve signals, leading to a wide range of symptoms, including numbness, weakness, vision issues, and cognitive impairment.

4. Psoriasis: Psoriasis is a chronic autoimmune disorder that mostly affects the skin, resulting in the fast proliferation of skin cells, and leading to the production of thick, red, scaly patches. In addition to skin symptoms, psoriasis can also damage the joints, causing a form of arthritis called psoriatic arthritis.

5. Celiac Disease: Celiac disease is an autoimmune illness produced by the intake of gluten, a protein found in wheat, barley, and rye. In individuals with celiac disease, gluten ingestion leads to damage to the small intestine, leading to symptoms such as abdominal pain, bloating, diarrhea, and loss of nutrients.

6. Type 1 Diabetes: Type 1 diabetes is an autoimmune disease defined by the loss of insulin-producing beta cells in the pancreas. This damage leads to insulin insufficiency, resulting in elevated blood sugar levels and the requirement for lifelong insulin therapy.

7. Hashimoto's Thyroiditis: Hashimoto's thyroiditis is an autoimmune illness that affects the thyroid gland, leading to inflammation and eventual death of thyroid tissue. This can result in hypothyroidism, marked by symptoms such as fatigue, weight gain, cold intolerance, and sadness.

Importance of Nutrition in Managing Autoimmune Conditions

Nutrition has a significant role in the management of autoimmune disorders, as it directly affects immune function, inflammation, and general health.

For individuals living with autoimmune diseases, adopting a nutrient-rich diet can be a significant aid in controlling symptoms, lowering inflammation, and promoting healing.

The Impact on Quality of Life

The impact of autoimmune disorders on a person's quality of life cannot be emphasized. Chronic pain, exhaustion, incapacity, and unpredictable symptom flare-ups can greatly limit daily functioning and affect overall well-being. Many patients with autoimmune disorders struggle to keep working, engage in social activities, and do ordinary duties due to the devastating nature of their symptoms.

Furthermore, the emotional toll of living with a chronic illness can lead to feelings of loneliness, frustration, and sadness. Coping with the physical limits and uncertainty associated with autoimmune disorders can have a considerable toll on mental health and interpersonal connections. Therefore, finding effective techniques for managing symptoms and enhancing quality of life is vital for persons living with autoimmune disorders.

The Role of the Immune System

The immune system functions as the body's defensive mechanism, protecting against outside invaders such as bacteria, viruses, and other infections. In patients with autoimmune illnesses, however, this defensive system becomes dysregulated, leading to the generation of autoantibodies that attack healthy tissues and organs.

The actual mechanisms behind autoimmune illnesses are complex and multifaceted, comprising a combination of genetic susceptibility, environmental variables, and dysregulated immune responses.

While researchers continue to understand the nuances of autoimmune illnesses, it is known that the immune system plays a major role in their genesis and progression.

How Food Affects the Immune System

Dietary choices can have a tremendous impact on immunological function and inflammation, both of which are major components of autoimmune disorders. Certain foods and dietary patterns have been proven to either increase or alleviate autoimmune symptoms, underscoring the relevance of nutrition in controlling these illnesses.

Meals That Promote Inflammation: Processed meals, refined carbohydrates, trans fats, and excessive consumption of red meat have been related to increased inflammation in the body. These foods can provoke immunological reactions and increase symptoms in individuals with autoimmune illnesses.

Foods That Reduce Inflammation: On the other hand, a diet rich in whole, unprocessed foods, including fruits, vegetables, whole grains, lean meats, and healthy fats, can help reduce inflammation and boost immunological function. These foods are filled with critical nutrients, antioxidants, and anti-inflammatory chemicals that can help alleviate the symptoms of autoimmune illnesses.

Specific Nutrients and Their Role: Certain nutrients play crucial roles in influencing immune function and inflammation. For example, omega-3 fatty acids found in fatty fish, flaxseeds, and walnuts have been demonstrated to lower inflammation and enhance cardiovascular health. Similarly, vitamin D, found in fatty fish, fortified dairy products, and sunlight exposure, plays a critical role in immune modulation and may help avoid autoimmune illnesses.

The Gut-Immune System Connection: The gut microbiome, comprised of billions of bacteria, fungi, and other microorganisms, plays a crucial role in immune function and inflammation. Emerging research suggests that dysbiosis, or imbalances in the gut microbiome, can contribute to the development and progression of autoimmune disorders. Therefore, maintaining a healthy gut microbiota by dietary treatments such as ingesting probiotic-rich foods, prebiotic fiber, and fermented foods may help boost immunological health and reduce inflammation. By adding anti-inflammatory, nutrient-dense foods t

o their meals and removing trigger foods, individuals can boost their immune systems, lessen symptoms, and improve their quality of life. Additionally, maintaining gut health with probiotic and prebiotic foods can further increase immune function and lower the likelihood of autoimmune flare-ups. Overall, a balanced and nutritious diet is vital for treating autoimmune illnesses and promoting health and well-being.

Chapter 1

The Science Behind Autoimmunity

Autoimmunity is a complicated and multidimensional phenomenon that emerges from dysfunction of the immune system. In healthy humans, the immune system serves as the body's defensive mechanism, protecting against outside invaders such as bacteria, viruses, and other diseases. However, in individuals with autoimmune diseases, this defense system becomes overactive and mistakenly assaults the body's own tissues and organs.

The Immune System Explained

The immune system is formed of a complex network of organs, tissues, cells, and chemicals that work together to defend the body against outside invaders and maintain homeostasis. Key components of the immune system include:

White Blood Cells: White blood cells, also known as leukocytes, are the fundamental biological components of the immune system.

They include lymphocytes (such as T cells and B cells), neutrophils, monocytes, eosinophils, and basophils, each with specialized roles in immune defense.

Lymphoid Organs: Lymphoid organs, such as the thymus, spleen, lymph nodes, and bone marrow, serve as locations for the generation and maturation of immune cells and the start of immunological responses.

Antibodies: Antibodies, also known as immunoglobulins, are proteins produced by B cells in response to certain antigens. They recognize and bind to foreign chemicals, marking them for destruction by other immune cells.

Cytokines: Cytokines are signaling molecules produced by immune cells that govern immunological responses and inflammation.

They include interleukins, interferons, tumor necrosis factors, and chemokines, among others.

Basics of Immune Function

The immune system acts through a complicated series of interactions and responses aimed at recognizing and destroying infections while sparing healthy tissues. Key components of immunological function include:

Identification: The immune system recognizes foreign invaders through the identification of certain molecular patterns known as antigens. Antigens might be proteins, carbohydrates, lipids, or other compounds found on the surface of pathogens.

Activation: Upon identification of antigens, the immune system mounts an immunological response, which comprises the activation and proliferation of immune cells, generation of antibodies, and release of cytokines.

Effector Mechanisms: Effector mechanisms of the immune response include phagocytosis (engulfment and destruction of pathogens by phagocytes), cytotoxicity (killing of infected or abnormal cells by cytotoxic T cells and natural killer cells), and antibody-mediated immunity (destruction of pathogens by antibodies).

Regulation: The immune system is strictly regulated to prevent excessive or inappropriate immune responses that can lead to tissue damage and autoimmune disorders. Regulatory mechanisms include the inhibition of immune cells, the creation of anti-inflammatory cytokines, and the induction of tolerance to self-antigens.

How the Immune System Works

The immune system functions through a sequence of synchronized actions aimed at identifying, neutralizing, and removing infections while limiting damage to healthy tissues. The process begins with the identification of foreign antigens by immune cells, such as dendritic cells, macrophages, and B cells. These cells subsequently present the antigens to T cells, which play a vital role in coordinating immunological responses.

Upon activation, T cells develop into effector T cells, such as cytotoxic T cells and helper T cells, which mediate distinct components of the immune response. Cytotoxic T cells identify and kill infected or aberrant cells, while helper T cells assist in the activation of other immune cells and the manufacture of antibodies by B cells.

Meanwhile, B cells differentiate into plasma cells, which manufacture antibodies specific to the antigen encountered. Antibodies bind to the antigen, designating it for destruction by other immune cells or neutralizing its effects. In addition to antibody-mediated immunity, the immune system also employs innate immunological processes, such as phagocytosis and inflammation, to eradicate pathogens.

Throughout the immune response, regulatory systems ensure that the immune system stays balanced and controlled, limiting excessive or inappropriate responses. These regulatory mechanisms include the action of regulatory T cells, the creation of anti-inflammatory cytokines, and the induction of tolerance to self-antigens. the immune system is a highly sophisticated and finely tuned network of cells, tissues, and chemicals that work together to protect the body against infection and preserve homeostasis. Dysregulation of the immune system can lead to autoimmune illnesses, where the body's tissues are mistakenly targeted and attacked. Understanding the foundations of immune function is vital for unraveling the intricacies of autoimmune disorders and finding effective treatments and interventions for people affected.

The Breakdown in Autoimmune Diseases

Autoimmune illnesses are defined by a failure in the body's immunological tolerance mechanisms, resulting in an inappropriate immune response against self-tissues and organs. Normally, the immune system distinguishes between self and non-self-antigens, targeting foreign invaders while protecting healthy tissues. However, in autoimmune illnesses, this self-tolerance mechanism fails, resulting in the development of autoantibodies and immune cells that attack the body's own cells and tissues.

What Goes Wrong with Autoimmune Disorders

In autoimmune illnesses, the immune system wrongly perceives the body's cells and tissues as alien or harmful, leading to an immune response directed against them. This might result in inflammation, tissue damage, and dysfunction of the affected organs or tissues. The specific mechanisms underlying autoimmune illnesses differ based on the ailment and the organs or tissues involved. For example:

In rheumatoid arthritis, the immune system targets the synovial membrane lining the joints, resulting in inflammation, discomfort, and damage to cartilage and bone.

In multiple sclerosis, the immune system targets the myelin sheath wrapping nerve fibers in the brain and spinal cord, interrupting nerve communication and leading to neurological symptoms.

In type 1 diabetes, the immune system destroys the insulin-producing beta cells in the pancreas, resulting in insulin insufficiency and elevated blood sugar levels.

These are just a few instances of the vast array of autoimmune illnesses and the mechanisms behind their development. In general, autoimmune illnesses are characterized by dysregulated immune responses, abnormal activation of immune cells, and generation of autoantibodies that target self-antigens.

Why Autoimmune Diseases Are on the Rise

Autoimmune illnesses are on the rise worldwide, with growing prevalence and incidence documented in recent decades. Several reasons contribute to this trend:

1. Environmental Changes: Environmental factors such as exposure to pollutants, poisons, infectious agents, and dietary changes have been implicated in the increase of autoimmune illnesses. Industrialization, urbanization, and changes in lifestyle and food have transformed the microbiological and chemical environments to which individuals are exposed, potentially causing or exacerbating autoimmune responses.

2. Changes in Hygiene Practices: The hygiene hypothesis posits that reduced exposure to viruses and microbial agents early in development may lead to dysregulated immune responses and greater vulnerability to autoimmune disorders. Improved sanitation, hygiene practices, and use of medicines have reduced exposure to infections, affecting the development and function of the immune system.

3. Western Diet: The Western diet, defined by a high intake of processed foods, refined sugars, saturated fats, and a low intake of fruits, vegetables, and fiber, has been related to an elevated risk of autoimmune illnesses. Poor eating habits can increase inflammation, dysbiosis (imbalance in the gut microbiota), and dysfunction of the immune system, contributing to the development of autoimmune disorders.

4. Genetic Predisposition: Genetic factors play a crucial role in the development of autoimmune illnesses, with specific genetic variants predisposing individuals to autoimmune susceptibility. However, genetic predisposition alone is not sufficient to produce autoimmune illnesses, and environmental stimuli are often necessary to initiate and prolong autoimmune responses.

Genetic and Environmental Factors

Autoimmune illnesses originate from a complicated interplay between genetic predisposition and environmental variables. While hereditary factors contribute to susceptibility to autoimmune illnesses, environmental triggers play a vital role in beginning and sustaining autoimmune responses. Several genetic risk factors have been identified for autoimmune illnesses, including particular gene variations involved with immune system control, antigen presentation, and cytokine signaling pathways.

However, the presence of these genetic risk factors alone is not sufficient to produce autoimmune illnesses, and environmental triggers are necessary to activate and worsen autoimmune responses. Environmental factors such as infections, nutritional factors, chemicals, pollutants, and stressors can induce or worsen autoimmune responses by modifying immune function, increasing inflammation, and affecting immunological tolerance mechanisms.

Genetic Link Between Cancer and Autoimmunity

The link between cancer and autoimmunity is complex and multifaceted, with accumulating evidence showing a similar genetic origin and overlapping immune dysregulation pathways. While cancer and autoimmune illnesses are separate clinical entities, they both include dysregulated immune responses and abnormal cellular mechanisms that might contribute to disease genesis and progression.

Genetic Factors: Genetic predisposition plays a crucial role in both cancer and autoimmune illnesses, with particular genetic variants associated with greater vulnerability to these conditions. Genomc-wide association studies (GWAS) have discovered common genetic risk factors shared between cancer and autoimmune illnesses, including genes implicated in immunological control, inflammation, and cellular proliferation.

Immune Dysregulation: Both cancer and autoimmune illnesses involve dysregulated immune responses characterized by abnormal activation or inhibition of immune cells and cytokines. In cancer, immune evasion mechanisms allow tumor cells to escape immune surveillance and proliferate unchecked. In autoimmune illnesses, dysregulated immune responses lead to the development of autoantibodies and inflammation, resulting in tissue damage and dysfunction.

Autoimmune Paraneoplastic Syndromes: Autoimmune paraneoplastic syndromes are a set of rare autoimmune illnesses that develop in conjunction with cancer. These disorders are hypothesized to develop from an immune response directed against common antigens produced by tumor cells and normal tissues. Examples of autoimmune paraneoplastic disorders include paraneoplastic pemphigus, dermatomyositis, and paraneoplastic cerebellar degeneration.

Treatment Implications: The connection between cancer and autoimmunity has substantial implications for cancer therapy and autoimmune disease management. Some cancer medications, such as immune checkpoint inhibitors, can provoke autoimmune reactions by boosting immune responses against tumor cells. Conversely, certain autoimmune illnesses may raise the chance of cancer development, demanding careful monitoring and therapy of both conditions.

Nutritional Science for Autoimmunity

Nutritional science plays a vital role in the management of autoimmune illnesses, giving prospective therapeutic options to control immune function, reduce inflammation, and improve overall health and well-being. While drugs and other traditional therapies are generally important for treating symptoms and preventing disease progression, dietary changes can complement existing approaches and provide extra benefits for persons living with autoimmune illnesses.

Macronutrients and Micronutrients Overview

Macronutrients: Macronutrients are the essential nutrients required by the body in significant amounts to support energy production, development, and metabolism. They contain carbs, proteins, and lipids, each of which serves a specific role in sustaining good health and immunological function.

Carbohydrates: Carbohydrates are the major source of energy for the body and play a critical function in fueling immune cells and sustaining general metabolism. Complex carbs, such as whole grains, fruits, and vegetables, give continuous energy and fiber, while simple carbohydrates, such as refined sugars and processed meals, should be consumed in moderation to avoid increases in blood sugar levels and inflammation.

Proteins: Proteins are the building blocks of tissues, organs, enzymes, and antibodies, making them crucial for immunological function and tissue healing. High-quality sources of protein, such as lean meats, poultry, fish, eggs, dairy products, legumes, nuts, and seeds, should be included in the diet to guarantee appropriate protein consumption and maintain immunological health.

Fats: Fats are vital for energy storage, hormone production, cell membrane integrity, and the absorption of fat-soluble vitamins. Healthy fats, such as monounsaturated and polyunsaturated fats found in olive oil, avocados, nuts, seeds, and fatty fish, have anti-inflammatory effects and can help reduce inflammation and promote immunological function.

Micronutrients: Micronutrients are necessary vitamins and minerals required by the body in lower amounts to support numerous physiological activities, including immunological function, antioxidant defense, and enzyme functioning. Key micronutrients for autoimmune health include:

Vitamin D: Vitamin D plays a vital function in immune modulation and has been linked to the development and progression of autoimmune disorders. Adequate vitamin

D levels are related to a lower risk of autoimmune disorders and improved disease outcomes.

Vitamin C: Vitamin C is a effective antioxidant that helps neutralize free radicals and minimize oxidative stress. It also enhances immunological function by boosting the development and function of immune cells, such as T cells and phagocytes.

Omega-3 Fatty Acids: Omega-3 fatty acids, found in fatty fish, flaxseeds, chia seeds, and walnuts, have anti-inflammatory qualities and can help reduce inflammation and improve immunological health. They also play a role in maintaining cell membrane integrity and influencing immune cell function.

Zinc: Zinc is an essential mineral that involves in immune function, wound healing, and DNA synthesis. Adequate zinc levels are crucial for effective immune cell activity and resistance against infections.

Selenium: Selenium is a trace mineral with antioxidant capabilities that helps protect against oxidative stress and inflammation. It also improves immunological function by boosting the activity of immune cells and lowering inflammation.

Anti-inflammatory Foods and Their Benefits

Inflammation is a significant cause of autoimmune disorders, contributing to tissue damage, discomfort, and dysfunction. Therefore, integrating anti-inflammatory foods into the diet can help reduce inflammation, alleviate symptoms, and improve general health and well-being. Some of the top anti-inflammatory foods include:

Fatty Fish: Fatty fish such as salmon, mackerel, sardines, and trout are rich in omega-3 fatty acids, which have significant anti-inflammatory qualities. Consuming fatty fish consistently can help reduce inflammation and improve immunological function.

Leafy Greens: Leafy green vegetables such as spinach, kale, Swiss chard, and collard greens are filled with vitamins, minerals, and phytochemicals that help battle inflammation and promote immunological function.

Berries: Berries such as blueberries, strawberries, raspberries, and blackberries are rich in antioxidants, including flavonoids and polyphenols, which help neutralize free radicals and reduce inflammation.

Nuts and Seeds: Nuts and seeds such as almonds, walnuts, flaxseeds, chia seeds, and hemp seeds are wonderful sources of healthy fats, fiber, and antioxidants. They provide anti-inflammatory elements like omega-3 fatty acids and vitamin E, which help reduce inflammation and boost immunological function.

Turmeric and Ginger: Turmeric and ginger are strong anti-inflammatory herbs that have been used for ages in traditional medicine. They contain bioactive chemicals such as curcumin and gingerol, which have potent anti-inflammatory and antioxidant activities.

Green Tea: Green tea is rich in polyphenols, particularly epigallocatechin gallate (EGCG), which has powerful anti-inflammatory and antioxidant properties. Drinking green tea consistently can help reduce inflammation and improve immunological function.

Healthy Oils: Healthy oils such as olive oil, avocado oil, and coconut oil are rich in monounsaturated and polyunsaturated fats, which have anti-inflammatory qualities. They also include antioxidants such as vitamin E and polyphenols, which help reduce inflammation and oxidative stress.

Fruits and Vegetables: Fruits and vegetables are rich in vitamins, minerals, antioxidants, and fiber, making them key components of an anti-inflammatory diet. Eating a range of colored fruits and vegetables can help reduce inflammation, support immunological function, and enhance overall health and well-being.

Incorporating these anti-inflammatory items into your diet can help reduce inflammation, alleviate symptoms, and boost immunological health in individuals with autoimmune illnesses. However, it's crucial to note that dietary modifications alone may not be adequate to control autoimmune illnesses, and they should be used in conjunction with other treatments and therapies as part of a comprehensive care plan.

Foods to Avoid and Why

In addition to including anti-inflammatory foods in your diet, it's also crucial to avoid or limit items that can aggravate inflammation and worsen symptoms in those with autoimmune illnesses. Some top inflammatory foods to avoid are:

Processed Foods: Processed foods such as fast food, packaged snacks, sweet desserts, and refined grains are generally high in harmful fats, sugars, and additives, which can promote inflammation and contribute to autoimmune symptoms.

Refined Sugars: Refined sugars such as table sugar, high-fructose corn syrup, and other sweeteners are readily absorbed into the system, causing spikes in blood sugar levels and increasing inflammation. Limiting intake of sugary foods and beverages can help reduce inflammation and improve immunological health.

Trans Fats: Trans fats, also known as partly hydrogenated oils, are chemically created fats found in fried foods, baked goods, margarine, and processed snacks. They are extremely inflammatory and can contribute to chronic inflammation and autoimmune disorders.

Dairy Products: Dairy products such as milk, cheese, and yogurt include proteins such as casein and whey, which might stimulate immunological responses in some people and exacerbate autoimmune symptoms. Lactose, the sugar present in dairy products, can also cause stomach difficulties in some people.

Gluten: Gluten is a protein found in wheat, barley, rye, and similar cereals. For individuals with gluten sensitivity or celiac disease, gluten consumption can provoke immunological responses and inflammation, leading to autoimmune symptoms and digestive issues.

Nightshade Vegetables: Nightshade vegetables such as tomatoes, peppers, eggplants, and potatoes contain substances called alkaloids, which can worsen inflammation and joint discomfort in some patients with autoimmune illnesses such as rheumatoid arthritis.

Avoiding these inflammatory foods can help reduce inflammation, alleviate symptoms, and enhance general health and well-being in those with autoimmune illnesses. However, it's vital to talk with a healthcare practitioner or qualified dietitian before making large dietary changes, especially if you have certain dietary limitations or medical issues.

Chapter 2

Dietary Strategies for Managing Autoimmune Diseases

Dietary procedures play an important function in controlling autoimmune diseases, offering a natural and alternative approach to traditional treatments. While drugs can help control symptoms and halt disease progression, dietary treatments can address underlying immunological dysregulation, reduce inflammation, and enhance general health and well-being. Two popular dietary treatments for addressing autoimmune illnesses are the elimination diet and the autoimmune protocol (AIP) diet.

The Elimination Diet

The elimination diet is a treatment technique that involves removing potential trigger foods from the diet and then carefully returning them to detect and eliminate food sensitivities or intolerances. The objective of the elimination diet is to identify and eliminate foods that may be contributing to inflammation, autoimmune symptoms, and immunological dysregulation.

Purpose and Plan

The objective of the elimination diet is to identify and eliminate potential trigger foods that may be worsening autoimmune symptoms or contributing to immune dysregulation. The approach often entails avoiding popular inflammatory foods for some time, such as 4-6 weeks, and then returning them one at a time while monitoring for symptoms.

The elimination phase of the diet often involves removing items that are known to be common triggers for food sensitivities or intolerances, such as gluten, dairy, soy, eggs, maize, nuts, seeds, nightshade vegetables, and processed foods. During this phase, individuals focus on consuming full, nutrient-dense foods such as fruits, vegetables, lean proteins, and healthy fats.

How to Implement Safely

When executing the elimination diet, it's especially important to do so safely and under the advice of a healthcare practitioner or certified dietitian. Here are some guidelines for executing the elimination diet safely:

Consult with a healthcare practitioner or certified dietitian before starting the elimination diet to confirm it is appropriate for your unique needs and health state.

Keep a food diary to note your symptoms and food intake during the elimination phase of the diet. This can help detect patterns and potential trigger foods.

Gradually reintroduce eliminated foods one at a time, in small quantities, and watch for any unpleasant reactions or symptoms. Pay attention to the changes in energy levels, digestion, mood, and overall well-being.

Reintroduce each food category separately and allow a few days between reintroductions to assess for delayed reactions.

Be patient and listen to your body. It may take time to
identify trigger foods and establish their impact on your
symptoms.

The Autoimmune Protocol (AIP) Diet

The autoimmune protocol (AIP) diet is a version of the
elimination diet specifically designed for patients with
autoimmune illnesses. It focuses on avoiding potential
trigger foods, lowering inflammation, and supporting gut
health to help manage autoimmune symptoms and
enhance overall well-being.

The AIP diet builds upon the concepts of the elimination
diet but takes a more comprehensive approach by
omitting additional foods that may contribute to immune
dysregulation or exacerbate autoimmune symptoms. In
addition to avoiding popular inflammatory foods, such as
gluten, dairy, soy, eggs, maize, nuts, seeds, and
processed foods, the AIP diet also excludes additional
foods that are known to be common triggers for
individuals with autoimmune illnesses.

Principles and Practices

When it comes to controlling autoimmune disorders with dietary treatments, various ideas and practices are routinely applied to enhance health outcomes and reduce symptoms. These ideas concentrate on strengthening immunological function, lowering inflammation, and promoting overall well-being. Some essential beliefs and behaviors include:

Nutrient Density: Emphasizing nutrient-dense meals that supply important vitamins, minerals, antioxidants, and phytochemicals is fundamental for maintaining immune function and general health. Prioritizing complete foods such as fruits, vegetables, lean proteins, healthy fats, and whole grains ensures a broad array of nutrients that support immunological health and minimize inflammation.

Anti-inflammatory Foods: Incorporating foods with anti-inflammatory qualities can help reduce inflammation and improve autoimmune symptoms. Anti-inflammatory foods include fatty fish rich in omega-3 fatty acids, leafy greens, berries, nuts, seeds, turmeric, ginger, and green tea. These foods have chemicals that assist modify immune responses and reduce inflammation.

Gut Health: Supporting gut health is vital for patients with autoimmune illnesses, as the gut flora plays a crucial role in immune regulation and inflammation. Consuming probiotic-rich foods such as yogurt, kefir, sauerkraut, and kimchi, as well as prebiotic-rich foods such as garlic, onions, and asparagus, can help maintain a healthy balance of gut flora and promote immune function.

Tailored Approach: Recognizing that autoimmune illnesses vary widely in their presentation and underlying processes, taking a tailored approach to nutritional management is necessary. What works for one person may not work for another, so it's crucial to adjust dietary advice to each person's distinct needs, preferences, and health goals.

Consistency and Patience: Consistency is crucial when it comes to dietary therapy for autoimmune illnesses. It may take time to see major improvements in symptoms, so patience and endurance are key. Making sustainable lifestyle adjustments and sticking to them over the long run can provide enduring benefits for immunological health and overall well-being.

Other Therapeutic Diets

In addition to the elimination diet and the autoimmune protocol (AIP) diet, various other therapeutic diets have been explored and applied in the management of autoimmune illnesses. These diets vary in their techniques and food restrictions but share the common goal of lowering inflammation, strengthening immune function, and enhancing the quality of life for patients with autoimmune illnesses. Some of the other therapeutic diets often utilized include:

Low-FODMAP Diet: The low-FODMAP diet is a dietary plan that restricts particular types of carbohydrates known as fermentable oligosaccharides, disaccharides, monosaccharides, and polyols

(FODMAPs). This diet is typically used to address gastrointestinal symptoms such as bloating, gas, and diarrhea in persons with disorders such as irritable bowel syndrome (IBS) and inflammatory bowel disease (IBD), which may coexist with autoimmune diseases.

Specific Carbohydrate Diet (SCD): The specific carbohydrate diet (SCD) is a dietary regimen that excludes complex carbs such as grains, dairy, and some sweets. It promotes nutrient-dense foods such as meats, seafood, eggs, fruits, vegetables, nuts, and seeds. SCD is widely used to control symptoms of gastrointestinal illnesses such as Crohn's disease, ulcerative colitis, and celiac disease, which may be connected with autoimmune diseases.

Low-Histamine Diet: The low-histamine diet restricts foods that are high in histamine or that may induce the release of histamine in the body. Histamine is a molecule implicated in immunological reactions and inflammation, and some individuals may be sensitive to high quantities of histamine in meals. The low-histamine diet is often used to address symptoms such as headaches, rashes, itching, and digestive difficulties in persons with histamine intolerance or mast cell activation syndrome.

Gluten-Free Diet: The gluten-free diet eliminates gluten, a protein found in wheat, barley, rye, and similar grains, from the diet. This diet is often used to control celiac disease, an autoimmune disorder characterized by an immunological sensitivity to gluten. Some persons with non-celiac gluten sensitivity or other autoimmune illnesses may also benefit from a gluten-free diet.

While these therapeutic diets may give comfort to some individuals with autoimmune illnesses, they may not be appropriate or successful for everyone. It's crucial to engage with a healthcare practitioner or registered dietitian to find the most effective nutritional approach for your unique needs and health goals.

Paleo, Vegan, and Ketogenic Approaches

The paleo, vegan, and ketogenic diets are three popular dietary regimens that have attracted attention for their possible health benefits, including their impact on inflammation, immunological function, and metabolic health. While these diets differ in their macronutrient composition and food selections, they share certain characteristics with therapeutic diets for autoimmune illnesses and may offer potential benefits for some individuals.

Paleo Diet: The paleo diet is based on the notion of consuming foods that our ancestors would have consumed during the Paleolithic era, such as lean meats, fish, fruits, vegetables, nuts, and seeds while avoiding processed foods, grains, dairy, and legumes. The paleo diet emphasizes natural, nutrient-dense foods and avoids processed foods and refined sugars, which can contribute to inflammation and autoimmune symptoms.

Vegan Diet: The vegan diet excludes all animal products and focuses on plant-based foods such as fruits, vegetables, grains, legumes, nuts, and seeds. While some research suggests that vegan diets may have anti-inflammatory effects and reduce the risk of chronic diseases, including autoimmune diseases, vegans need to ensure they are meeting their nutrient needs, particularly for essential nutrients such as protein, iron, calcium, vitamin B12, and omega-3 fatty acids.

Ketogenic Diet: The ketogenic diet is a high-fat, low-carbohydrate diet that has gained popularity for its potential benefits in weight loss, metabolic health, and neurological diseases such as epilepsy. The ketogenic diet increases the generation of ketones, which are alternate fuel sources for the brain and body when glucose levels are low. Some data suggest that the ketogenic diet may have anti-inflammatory benefits and reduce symptoms in patients with autoimmune illnesses, although further studies are needed to completely understand its impact.

Comparative Analysis and Personalization

When comparing therapeutic diets such as the elimination diet, the AIP diet, and other nutritional approaches such as paleo, vegan, and ketogenic diets, it's crucial to assess their specific strengths, limitations, and applicability for persons with autoimmune illnesses. Each diet has its distinct principles, food limits, and potential benefits, which may vary depending on an individual's personal health condition, preferences, and goals.

Comparative Analysis:

Elimination Diet vs. AIP Diet: Both the elimination diet and the AIP diet strive to identify and eliminate trigger foods that may increase autoimmune symptoms and inflammation. However, the AIP diet is more stringent than the elimination diet, as it excludes additional items such as nightshade vegetables, eggs, nuts, and seeds, which are significant triggers for patients with autoimmune illnesses. The AIP diet also emphasizes gut health and includes guidelines for lifestyle aspects such as stress management and sleep hygiene. While both diets may provide symptom alleviation for some individuals, the AIP diet may be more beneficial for those with severe autoimmune symptoms or numerous autoimmune disorders.

Paleo Diet vs. Vegan Diet: The paleo diet and the vegan diet differ greatly in their food choices and macronutrient makeup. The paleo diet emphasizes full, nutrient-dense foods such as lean meats, fish, fruits, vegetables, nuts, and seeds while excluding processed foods, grains, dairy, and legumes. In contrast, the vegan diet excludes all animal products and emphasizes plant-based foods such as fruits, vegetables, grains, legumes, nuts, and seeds. While these diets may have anti-inflammatory effects and reduce the risk of chronic diseases, persons with autoimmune diseases may need to alter these diets to ensure they meet their nutrient needs and support immune function sufficiently.

Ketogenic Diet vs. Other Therapeutic Diets: The ketogenic diet varies from other therapeutic diets in its macronutrient composition and metabolic consequences. While the ketogenic diet is high in fat and low in carbs, other therapeutic diets such as the elimination diet, the AIP diet, and the paleo diet focus on complete, nutrient-dense meals and may include carbohydrates from fruits, vegetables, and whole grains. Some research suggests that the ketogenic diet may have anti-inflammatory benefits and reduce symptoms in patients with autoimmune illnesses, but further studies are needed to properly understand its long-term impact and safety.

Personalization:

Personalizing dietary therapy for individuals with autoimmune illnesses is critical to enhance health outcomes and improve quality of life. Factors such as individual health status, medical history, dietary preferences, cultural background, and lifestyle factors should be taken into consideration when designing a tailored dietary plan. A personalized approach may involve:

Full examination: Conducting a full examination of an individual's health status, including their autoimmune condition, symptoms, medical history, nutritional status, dietary habits, and lifestyle factors, is necessary for designing a personalized dietary plan.

Collaboration with Healthcare Professionals:
Collaborating with healthcare professionals such as

physicians, registered dietitians, nutritionists, and other allied health professionals can provide valuable support and guidance in developing a personalized dietary plan tailored to an individual's specific needs and goals.

Trial and Error: Experimenting with different dietary methods and monitoring their effects on symptoms, energy levels, digestion, mood, and general well-being can help find the most successful dietary interventions for an individual with an autoimmune disease.

Long-run Maintenance: Establishing sustainable dietary habits and lifestyle modifications that can be sustained over the long run is vital for treating autoimmune illnesses and promoting general health and well-being. Regular monitoring and change of dietary patterns may be important to suit changing demands and enhance health results throughout time. numerous nutritional methods, including the elimination diet, the AIP diet, and other therapeutic diets such as paleo, vegan, and ketogenic diets, offer potential benefits for patients with autoimmune illnesses. Each diet has its distinct ideas, practices, and potential benefits, which should be carefully evaluated and adjusted to meet an individual's specific needs, preferences, and goals. By adopting a tailored approach to nutritional management and working together with healthcare providers, individuals with autoimmune illnesses can optimize health outcomes and improve quality of life.

Chapter 3

Meal Planning and Recipes

Meal planning is a critical element of controlling autoimmune illnesses through dietary therapy. By carefully selecting and preparing nutritious meals, individuals can support immune function, minimize inflammation, and promote general health and well-being. Here are some crucial aspects for good meal planning:

Building a Balanced Meal Plan

A balanced meal plan should include a range of nutrient-dense foods from all food groups to guarantee appropriate consumption of important nutrients. Aim to include:

Lean proteins such as poultry, fish, eggs, tofu, or lentils assist muscle function and repair.

Whole grains such as quinoa, brown rice, oats, or barley provide sustained energy and fiber.

Plenty of fruits and vegetables of different colors supply vitamins, minerals, antioxidants, and fiber.

Healthy fats from sources like avocados, nuts, seeds, olive oil, or fatty fish can boost brain function and prevent inflammation.

Dairy alternatives such as almond milk, coconut yogurt, or cashew cheese are available for people with dairy sensitivity.

Herbs, spices, and seasonings help add flavor and boost the nutritional content of meals without relying on excessive salt or sugar.

Portion Sizes and Frequency

Understanding portion sizes and meal frequency is vital for maintaining balanced nutrition and managing autoimmune symptoms. Aim to:

Eat regular meals and snacks throughout the day to maintain steady blood sugar levels and minimize energy dips.

Practice portion control by utilizing measuring cups, food scales, or visual cues to guarantee optimal serving sizes of different food groups.

Listen to your body's hunger and fullness cues to avoid overeating or undereating.

Consider dividing your plate into sections, with half filled with vegetables, a quarter with protein, and a quarter with grains or starchy vegetables to assist in visualizing balanced meals.

Ensuring Nutrient Diversity

Ensuring nutrient diversity is crucial to meeting your body's nutritional demands and promoting immunological function. Try to:

Incorporate a wide variety of foods from diverse food groups, colors, and textures into your meals and snacks.

Rotate your meal choices often to expose yourself to a broad spectrum of vitamins, minerals, antioxidants, and phytochemicals.

Experiment with different cooking methods, such as steaming, roasting, grilling, or sautéing, to boost flavor and nutrient bioavailability.

Consider introducing superfoods such as kale, spinach, berries, turmeric, ginger, garlic, and almonds into your meals and snacks for their tremendous health-promoting benefits.

Recipes for Health

Here are some simple and healthful recipes to inspire your meal planning:

Quinoa Salad: Cooked quinoa tossed with diced cucumber, cherry tomatoes, bell peppers, red onion, fresh herbs (such as parsley or cilantro), lemon juice, olive oil, salt, and pepper. Optional ingredients include avocado, feta cheese, grilled chicken, or chickpeas for extra protein.

Baked Salmon with Roasted Vegetables: Seasoned salmon fillets baked in the oven until flaky, served with a side of roasted vegetables (such as carrots, broccoli, and Brussels sprouts) coated in olive oil, garlic, herbs, salt, and pepper.

Vegetable Stir-Fry: Stir-fried mixed vegetables (such as bell peppers, snap peas, carrots, mushrooms, and broccoli) with tofu or shrimp in a flavorful sauce made from soy sauce (or tamari for gluten-free option), ginger, garlic, sesame oil, and a touch of honey or maple syrup, served over brown rice or quinoa.

Green Smoothie: Blend spinach, kale, banana, frozen berries, almond milk, Greek yogurt (or dairy-free yogurt replacement), and a scoop of protein powder (such as pea protein or collagen peptides) until smooth and creamy. Optional additions include chia seeds, flaxseeds, nut butter, or a handful of spinach for added nutrients.

These recipes are only a starting point for making delicious and healthy meals that boost immunological function and reduce autoimmune symptoms. Feel free to alter them based on your preferences, dietary restrictions, and nutritional needs. Experiment with varied products, flavors, and cooking techniques to keep your meals interesting and pleasurable while nourishing your body and encouraging overall well-being.

Breakfast, Lunch, and Dinner Ideas

Starting the day with a nutritious meal sets the tone for the rest of the day and provides the necessary fuel for energy and focus. Consider options such as:

Overnight Oats: Combine rolled oats with almond milk, chia seeds, Greek yogurt (or dairy-free substitute), and your choice of toppings such as berries, nuts, seeds, and a drizzle of honey or maple syrup. Let it sit in the refrigerator overnight, and have a handy and nutritious breakfast in the morning.

Vegetable Omelette: Whisk together eggs or egg whites with diced vegetables such as bell peppers, spinach, mushrooms, and onions. Cook in a non-stick skillet until set, then serve with a side of avocado slices and whole-grain bread or sweet potato hash.

Smoothie Bowl: Blend frozen fruits such as berries, bananas, and spinach with almond milk, Greek yogurt (or protein powder), and a handful of spinach or kale until smooth and creamy. Pour into a bowl and top with granola, nuts, seeds, and more fruit for added texture and flavor.

For lunch and dinner, focus on balanced meals that incorporate lean proteins, whole grains, healthy fats, and lots of vegetables:

Grilled Chicken Salad: Grilled chicken breast seasoned with herbs and spices and served over a bed of mixed greens with cherry tomatoes, cucumber slices, shredded carrots, avocado, and a sprinkle of balsamic vinaigrette. Add quinoa or brown rice on the side for extra nutrition and satiety.

Quinoa Stir-Fry: Stir-fry cooked quinoa with mixed veggies such as bell peppers, snap peas, broccoli, and tofu or shrimp in a savory sauce made from soy sauce (or tamari), ginger, garlic, sesame oil, and honey or maple syrup. Serving hot with a sprinkle of sesame seeds and chopped green onions.

Salmon with Roasted Vegetables: Bake salmon fillets seasoned with lemon, garlic, and herbs in the oven until flaky. Serve with a side of roasted vegetables such as Brussels sprouts, carrots, and sweet potatoes drizzled in olive oil, salt, and pepper.

Snacks and Desserts

Healthy snacks can help keep hunger at bay between meals and give additional nutrients and energy. Consider options such as:

Greek Yogurt with Berries: Enjoy a serving of Greek yogurt (or dairy-free option) topped with fresh berries, a drizzle of honey or maple syrup, and a sprinkling of nuts or seeds for extra crunch and protein.

Homemade Trail Mix: Mix a variety of nuts, seeds, and dried fruits such as almonds, cashews, pumpkin seeds, sunflower seeds, dried cranberries, and apricots for a delightful and nutrient-rich snack.

Apple Slices with Almond Butter: Spread almond butter on apple slices for a delightful and full snack that combines fiber, healthy fats, and natural sweetness.

For desserts, go for healthier alternatives that fulfill your sweet taste without compromising your health goals:

Dark Chocolate Bark: Melt dark chocolate and spread it onto a parchment-lined baking sheet. Top with chopped nuts, seeds, dried fruits, and a sprinkling of sea salt. Let it solidify in the refrigerator, then break it into pieces for a delectable and antioxidant-rich treat.

Frozen Banana Bites: Slice bananas into coins and dip them in melted dark chocolate. Place them on a parchment-lined baking sheet and freeze until hard. Enjoy as a refreshing and naturally sweet dessert or snack.

Chia Seed Pudding: Mix chia seeds with almond milk, a sprinkle of vanilla essence, and a touch of maple syrup or honey. Let it sit in the refrigerator for a few hours or overnight until it thickens. Serve with fresh fruit or a dollop of Greek yogurt for extra flavor and texture.

Tips for Meal Prep and Storage

Meal planning and storage can save time and simplify healthy eating throughout the week. Consider the following tips:

Plan Ahead: Take some time each week to plan your meals and snacks, create a shopping list, and prep ingredients in advance.

Batch Cooking: Cook large batches of grains, meats, and vegetables at the beginning of the week and portion them out into individual containers for convenient grab-and-go meals.

Use Proper Containers: Invest in quality storage containers that are freezer-safe, microwave-safe, and leak-proof to keep your meals fresh and prevent spillage.

Label and Date: Label your containers with the contents and date of preparation to keep track of freshness and minimize food waste.

Stock Up on Essentials: Keep your pantry stocked with fundamental goods such as grains, canned beans, nuts, seeds, spices, and sauces to make meal prep quicker and more convenient.

By implementing these meal planning and preparation tactics into your routine, you can streamline healthy eating, save time, and ensure you always have nutritious options on hand to support your health and well-being.

Superfoods for Autoimmune Health

Superfoods are nutrient-rich foods that are particularly useful for overall health and well-being, including strengthening immune function and lowering inflammation in individuals with autoimmune illnesses. Incorporating these superfoods into your diet can provide a wide range of vitamins, minerals, antioxidants, and phytochemicals that support immunological health and help control autoimmune symptoms. Some notable superfoods for autoimmune health include:

Turmeric, Ginger, and Garlic

Turmeric, ginger, and garlic are effective anti-inflammatory herbs and spices that have been used for millennia in traditional medicine for their healing effects.

Turmeric includes curcumin, a substance with potent anti-inflammatory and antioxidant properties. Ginger is recognized for its anti-inflammatory and digestive effects, while garlic possesses immune-boosting and antibacterial characteristics. Incorporating these spices into your meals can help reduce inflammation, support immunological function, and alleviate autoimmune symptoms.

Leafy Greens and Cruciferous Vegetables

Leafy greens such as spinach, kale, Swiss chard, and collard greens are filled with vitamins, minerals, antioxidants, and fiber that boost immune health and reduce inflammation. Cruciferous plants such as broccoli, cauliflower, Brussels sprouts, and cabbage contain sulfur compounds and phytochemicals that have anti-inflammatory and detoxifying benefits. Including a variety of leafy greens and cruciferous vegetables in your diet can help maintain gut health, assist liver detoxification, and modify immunological responses in those with autoimmune illnesses.

Fermented Foods and Probiotics

Fermented foods such as yogurt, kefir, sauerkraut, kimchi, and kombucha are high in helpful microorganisms known as probiotics. These probiotics assist in maintaining a healthy balance of gut bacteria, improve immunological function, and reduce inflammation in people with autoimmune illnesses. Consuming fermented foods consistently can assist improve digestion, promote nutrient absorption, and strengthen the gut barrier, which is critical for patients with autoimmune disorders because gut health plays a vital role in illness management.

Incorporating these superfoods into your diet can be as simple as adding turmeric and ginger to curries and stir-fries, incorporating leafy greens and cruciferous vegetables in salads and smoothies, and enjoying fermented foods as snacks or side dishes. By making these nutrient-rich foods a regular part of your diet, you may give your body the critical nutrients and chemicals it needs to promote immunological health, reduce inflammation, and manage autoimmune symptoms successfully.

Chapter 4

The Healing Power of Nutrition

Within the context of promoting health and healing, nutrition is an extremely important factor, particularly for people who suffer from autoimmune diseases. The ability of diet to supply critical nutrients that support immune function, reduce inflammation, and promote overall well-being is the source of the healing power of nutrition. To effectively manage autoimmune disorders, it is vital to have a diet that is well-balanced and places an emphasis on foods that are rich in nutrients. This diet can help control immune responses, support tissue repair, and optimize metabolic processes.

The Autoimmune Diet Paradigm

Identifying and removing foods that cause inflammation and increase autoimmune symptoms is the primary focus of the autoimmune diet paradigm. At the same time, nutrient-dense foods that promote immunological health and reduce inflammation are given priority. Through the avoidance of common allergens, food sensitivities, and inflammatory compounds, this dietary strategy seeks to restore equilibrium within the immune system and reduce the frequency of autoimmune flare-ups. The paradigm of the autoimmune diet typically consists of an elimination phase, which is then followed by a gradual reintroduction of foods. This methodology is utilized to identify specific triggers and develop a personalized dietary plan.

The Concept of Food as Medicine

Taking into account the fact that the foods we consume have a direct influence on our health and well-being, the concept of food as medicine acknowledges this fact. Certain foods have therapeutic properties that can assist in the prevention, management, and even reversal of chronic diseases, this includes ailments that are associated with the immune system. By electing nutrient-dense, whole foods that contain anti-inflammatory chemicals, antioxidants, and critical nutrients, individuals can harness the healing power of food to promote immune function, reduce inflammation, and enhance health outcomes.

Nutrient-Dense vs. Inflammatory Foods

Nutrient-dense foods have a high concentration of vital nutrients compared to their calorie level, making them valuable sources of vitamins, minerals, antioxidants, and phytochemicals. Examples of nutrient-dense foods include leafy greens, colorful vegetables, fruits, lean meats, nuts, seeds, and whole grains. These foods support immune function, reduce inflammation, and enhance general health and well-being.

In contrast, inflammatory foods are those that increase inflammation within the body and may exacerbate autoimmune symptoms. Common inflammatory foods include processed foods, refined sugars, trans fats, excessive alcohol, and foods heavy in sodium and saturated fats. These foods can contribute to immunological dysregulation, oxidative stress, and tissue damage, making them detrimental for those with autoimmune illnesses.

Understanding the distinction between nutrient-dense and inflammatory foods is vital for building an autoimmune-friendly diet that supports health and healing. By choosing nutrient-dense foods and avoiding inflammatory triggers, individuals can optimize their nutritional intake, reduce autoimmune symptoms, and improve their quality of life. Adopting a whole-foods-based diet that stresses the healing power of nutrition can be a revolutionary approach to treating autoimmune illnesses and supporting long-term health and well-being.

The Gut-Immune Connection

The gut-immune connection refers to the complicated interplay between the gut bacteria and the immune system. The gut houses trillions of microorganisms, including bacteria, fungi, and viruses, collectively known as the gut microbiota. These microorganisms serve a vital role in modulating immunological responses and maintaining immune homeostasis. The gut-associated lymphoid tissue (GALT), which is a fundamental component of the immune system, interacts closely with the gut microbiota to affect immune activity. Dysregulation of the gut-immune axis can lead to immunological dysfunction, inflammation, and the development or worsening of autoimmune disorders. Therefore, maintaining gut health through food and lifestyle treatments is critical for controlling autoimmune disorders and increasing overall immunological resilience.

Anti-Inflammatory Foods

Anti-inflammatory foods are those that help reduce inflammation in the body and promote immunological balance. Incorporating a range of anti-inflammatory items into your diet can help modify immune responses and reduce autoimmune symptoms. These foods often contain chemicals that inhibit inflammatory processes and promote tissue healing. By focusing on an anti-inflammatory diet, persons with autoimmune illnesses can better control their condition and improve overall health outcomes.

Highlighting Specific Foods with Anti-Inflammatory Properties

Several foods are known for their significant anti-inflammatory qualities and can be beneficial for patients with autoimmune illnesses. Some important instances include:

Turmeric: Contains curcumin, a strong anti-inflammatory substance that inhibits inflammatory enzymes and modifies immunological responses.

Ginger: Has natural anti-inflammatory and antioxidant qualities, which can help reduce pain and inflammation linked with autoimmune disorders.

Berries: Rich in antioxidants and phytochemicals that battle oxidative stress and inflammation in the body.

Fatty Fish: Such as salmon, mackerel, and sardines, are abundant in omega-3 fatty acids, which have significant anti-inflammatory properties.

Leafy Greens: Such as spinach, kale, and Swiss chard, are filled with vitamins, minerals, and antioxidants that boost immune health and reduce inflammation.

Incorporating Antioxidants, Omega-3 Fatty Acids, and Phytonutrients

Antioxidants, omega-3 fatty acids, and phytonutrients are vital components of an anti-inflammatory diet that supports immunological function and decreases inflammation. Antioxidants protect cells from oxidative stress and free radical damage, which are common contributors to inflammation and autoimmune disorders. Omega-3 fatty acids, notably EPA (eicosatetraenoic acid) and DHA (docosahexaenoic acid) found in fatty fish and flaxseeds, have significant anti-inflammatory characteristics and can help modify immunological responses. Phytonutrients, found in colored fruits, vegetables, and herbs, include bioactive components that boost immune function, reduce inflammation, and improve general health and well-being.

Incorporating these nutrients into your diet through full, nutrient-dense foods is vital for controlling autoimmune diseases and optimizing immunological health. By focusing on anti-inflammatory foods rich in antioxidants, omega-3 fatty acids, and phytonutrients, individuals can strengthen the gut-immune connection, reduce inflammation, and enhance immunological resilience in the setting of autoimmune illnesses. Adopting a balanced and diverse diet that promotes these nutrient-rich foods can play a crucial role in treating autoimmune symptoms and enhancing overall quality of life.

The Importance of a Colorful Plate

A colorful plate is not merely physically pleasing but also suggestive of a variety and nutrient-rich diet. Different colors of fruits and vegetables signify distinct phytonutrients, antioxidants, vitamins, and minerals that contribute to general health and immunological function. Incorporating a wide array of colors into meals guarantees a broad spectrum of nutrients, which can boost immunological modulation and reduce inflammation. For example, red and orange veggies like bell peppers and carrots are high in beta-carotene, while leafy greens like spinach and kale give critical vitamins such as folate and vitamin K. Including a spectrum of colors on your plate can assist improve food intake and boost immunological health in those with autoimmune illnesses.

Common Triggers: Gluten, Dairy, and Processed Sugars

Gluten, dairy, and processed sugars are prominent dietary factors that can aggravate inflammation and autoimmune symptoms in vulnerable individuals. Gluten, a protein found in wheat, barley, and rye, can stimulate immunological responses and contribute to gut inflammation in persons with gluten sensitivity or celiac disease. Dairy products contain proteins like casein and lactose that may induce inflammation and digestive difficulties in some individuals with lactose intolerance or dairy sensitivity. Processed sweets, including refined sugars and high-fructose corn syrup, can disturb gut flora, induce inflammation, and contribute to metabolic dysfunction. Avoiding these common triggers can help

minimize autoimmune flare-ups and improve overall
health.

Nightshades and Lectins

Nightshades (such as tomatoes, eggplants, peppers, and
potatoes) and lectins (found in beans, lentils, and grains)
are controversial foods that some people with
autoimmune illnesses prefer to avoid due to their
tendency to worsen inflammation and digestive
difficulties. Nightshades include alkaloids that may
cause inflammatory reactions in sensitive individuals,
while lectins are plant proteins that can attach to cells in
the stomach and potentially contribute to leaky gut and
immunological activation. However, the impact of
nightshades and lectins on autoimmune illnesses varies
greatly among individuals, and not everyone may need
to avoid these items from their diet.

Personalized investigation and observation can help
discover whether these foods are triggers for specific
autoimmune conditions.

Personalized Elimination Diets

Personalized elimination diets entail carefully removing suspected trigger foods from the diet and then returning them one at a time to identify specific dietary culprits that contribute to autoimmune symptoms. This strategy allows users to pinpoint which foods cause inflammation or immunological reactions and adapt their diet accordingly. Commonly removed foods on an elimination diet include gluten-containing cereals, dairy products, processed sweets, nightshades, lectin-containing foods, and other suspected allergies. Keeping a detailed food diary and documenting symptoms during the exclusion and reintroduction phases can help discover specific triggers and inform dietary alterations that promote autoimmune management and symptom relief.

The importance of a colorful plate lies in its ability to supply a varied array of nutrients that support immunological function and reduce inflammation. Common dietary irritants such as gluten, dairy, and processed sweets can worsen autoimmune symptoms and should be avoided or limited. Nightshades and lectins are controversial foods that may influence certain individuals with autoimmune illnesses, but their impact varies widely, necessitating tailored experimentation. Personalized elimination diets can assist in discovering particular dietary triggers and inform individualized dietary practices that promote autoimmune treatment and overall well-being.

Chapter 5

Navigating Challenges and Roadblocks

Managing autoimmune disorders can bring many hurdles and roadblocks that demand perseverance, adaptation, and determination. Understanding and resolving these obstacles is critical for effectively managing symptoms and promoting overall health and well-being.

Common Challenges Faced When Managing Autoimmune Conditions

Individuals with autoimmune disorders often experience many problems that can impair their ability to adhere to treatment plans and maintain a healthy lifestyle. Some common issues include unpredictable flare-ups of symptoms, exhaustion, pain, and limitations in physical activities. Dietary limitations and the need to avoid specific foods or food groups can often be hard, especially in social or cultural circumstances.

Additionally, negotiating complex treatment regimens, managing drug side effects, and dealing with mental stress and worry connected to the chronic nature of autoimmune disorders can offer substantial challenges to good health.

Strategies for Overcoming Obstacles and Maintaining Motivation

Overcoming issues connected with autoimmune disorders involves a multidimensional approach that addresses physical, emotional, and practical elements of health management. Strategies for overcoming hurdles and retaining motivation include:

Education and Awareness: Stay informed about your condition, treatment options, and lifestyle improvements that can help manage symptoms successfully.

Self-Care Practices: Prioritize self-care activities such as regular exercise, appropriate sleep, stress management techniques (e.g., meditation, yoga), and relaxation therapies to support general well-being.

Adaptive Lifestyle Modifications: Modify daily routines and activities to suit changing energy levels and physical restrictions caused by autoimmune symptoms.

Nutritional boost: Follow an anti-inflammatory diet customized to your unique needs, incorporating nutrient-dense foods that boost immune function and reduce inflammation.

Mindset and Resilience: Cultivate a positive mindset, practice self-compassion, and seek support from mental health specialists or support groups to cope with emotional issues associated with chronic illness.

Building a Support System for Your Health Journey

Building a solid support system is vital for overcoming the obstacles of managing autoimmune disorders. A supportive network of family members, friends, healthcare practitioners, and fellow individuals with autoimmune disorders can provide encouragement, practical assistance, and emotional support. Consider the following approaches to develop a support system for your health journey:

Communicate: Share your needs, concerns, and aspirations with trusted others who can offer empathy and understanding.

Seek Professional advice: Consult with healthcare specialists, including doctors, nutritionists, and counselors, who specialize in autoimmune illnesses and may provide specialized advice and support.

Join Support Groups: Connect with online or local support groups for those with autoimmune disorders to share experiences, discuss tips, and find solidarity.

Engage in Community Activities: Participate in community events, workshops, or programs relating to health and wellness to broaden your social network and locate like-minded folks.

By proactively addressing challenges, using effective techniques, and developing a supportive network, persons with autoimmune disorders can overcome obstacles, sustain motivation, and enhance their health journey for long-term well-being.

Chapter 6

Lifestyle Factors for Managing Autoimmune Disease

Managing autoimmune disease entails adopting healthy lifestyle habits that improve general well-being and immunological health. Lifestyle decisions can greatly impact disease development, symptom intensity, and quality of life for those with autoimmune disorders. Key lifestyle considerations for managing autoimmune illness include:

Nutrition: Following an anti-inflammatory diet rich in whole foods, fruits, vegetables, healthy fats, and lean proteins will help reduce inflammation and support immunological function.

Physical Activity: Regular exercise can improve cardiovascular health, build muscles, and reduce stress, which is useful for treating autoimmune symptoms.

Sleep: Prioritizing appropriate sleep and keeping a consistent sleep schedule can boost immune function, reduce inflammation, and promote general health.

Stress Management: Implementing stress-reduction practices such as mindfulness, meditation, and relaxation can help control immune responses and relieve autoimmune symptoms.

Importance of Stress Management in Autoimmune Health

Stress can aggravate autoimmune symptoms by activating inflammatory responses and altering immunological function. Chronic stress can contribute to immunological dysregulation, hormone abnormalities, and increased susceptibility to infections or flare-ups of autoimmune illnesses. Effective stress management is vital for maintaining immunological resilience and avoiding autoimmune symptoms. By incorporating stress-reduction measures into everyday routines, persons with autoimmune disorders can better manage stressors and improve overall health.

Mindfulness, Meditation, and Relaxation Techniques

Mindfulness, meditation, and relaxation practices are important strategies for reducing stress and enhancing emotional well-being in individuals with autoimmune illnesses. These techniques help foster present-moment awareness, reduce anxiety, and boost resilience to stress. Mindfulness techniques such as deep breathing exercises, body scans, and guided meditation can stimulate the body's relaxation response, which counteracts the negative effects of chronic stress on the immune system. Regular practice of mindfulness and meditation can improve emotional balance, strengthen coping skills, and support immunological function in patients with autoimmune disorders.

Prioritizing Self-Care

Prioritizing self-care is vital for those with autoimmune disorders to maintain physical, emotional, and mental well-being. Self-care activities involve caring for oneself and satisfying personal needs to boost general health and resilience. Some self-care practices for those with autoimmune illnesses include:

Setting Boundaries: Establishing healthy boundaries with job, social commitments, and personal relationships to avoid overexertion and decrease stress.

Engaging in Hobbies: Allocating time for fun activities and hobbies that encourage relaxation and bring a sense of fulfillment.

Seeking Support: Connecting with helpful persons, participating in support groups, or seeking professional counseling to address emotional difficulties and increase coping abilities.

Practicing Gratitude: Cultivating gratitude via everyday practices such as journaling or expressing appreciation for pleasant elements of life can increase emotional well-being and resilience.

By prioritizing self-care and adopting stress-reduction practices into daily routines, individuals with autoimmune disorders can enhance their quality of life, manage symptoms efficiently, and support overall immunological function. Adopting a holistic strategy that includes lifestyle variables, stress management, and self-care practices is crucial to maximizing health outcomes and fostering long-term well-being in the setting of autoimmune illnesses.

Sleep Hygiene

Sleep hygiene refers to a collection of behaviors and habits that support good sleep quality and quantity. Good sleep hygiene is critical for overall health and well-being, including immunological function and the management of autoimmune disorders. Adopting appropriate sleep practices can improve sleep efficiency, enhance immunological resilience, and support overall immune health.

Quality Sleep and Its Impact on Immune Function

Quality sleep plays a vital role in modulating immunological function and building immune resilience. During sleep, the body performs key activities that contribute to immune health, including the generation of immune cells and the release of cytokines that govern immune responses. Adequate and restorative sleep helps enhance immune function, reduce inflammation, and boost the body's capacity to fight off infections and manage autoimmune disorders successfully.

Establishing a Sleep Routine

Establishing a consistent sleep habit is crucial to ensuring quality sleep and supporting immunological function. A sleep pattern entails developing a disciplined plan for bedtime and wake-up time, as well as including relaxing activities to notify the body that it's time to wind down. Consistency is vital for regulating the body's internal clock and fostering healthy sleep. To establish a sleep routine:

Set a consistent bedtime and wake-up time, especially on weekends.

Create a pleasant pre-sleep ritual, such as reading a book, having a warm bath, or practicing relaxation techniques.

Avoid stimulating activities and screens (e.g., phones, computers, TVs) before bedtime.

Keep the bedroom environment favorable to sleep by having a comfortable mattress, suitable room temperature, and little noise and light.

Tips for Better Sleep Quality

Improving sleep quality entails adopting healthy habits and making adjustments to encourage peaceful and refreshing sleep. Some recommendations for greater sleep quality include:

Limiting caffeine and avoiding heavy meals, tobacco, and alcohol close to bedtime.

Creating a peaceful and dark sleep environment by employing blackout curtains and limiting noise interruptions.

Engaging in regular physical activity during the day but avoiding severe exercise close to nighttime.

Manage stress through relaxation methods such as deep breathing, meditation, or yoga.

Avoid napping late in the day, particularly if experiencing problems falling asleep at night.

Sleep hygiene, creating a consistent sleep regimen, and applying techniques for improving sleep quality, individuals with autoimmune illnesses can optimize immune function, manage symptoms efficiently, and promote overall health and well-being. Quality sleep is a cornerstone of immunological function and should be targeted as part of a holistic approach to managing autoimmune diseases.

The Role of Exercise and Physical Activity

Exercise and physical activity play a significant role in controlling autoimmune disorders by boosting immunological function, increasing cardiovascular health, enhancing muscle strength, and promoting general well-being. Regular exercise can help reduce inflammation, alleviate symptoms such as fatigue and joint pain, and enhance immunological resilience in patients with autoimmune illnesses. However, it's crucial to adjust exercise programs to individual requirements and capabilities to avoid worsening symptoms or causing injury.

Gentle Exercises for Autoimmune Patients

For patients with autoimmune illnesses, gentle workouts that emphasize low-impact motions and flexibility are generally prescribed to avoid strain on joints and muscles while developing mobility and strength. Examples of gentle activities good for autoimmune patients include:

Yoga: Incorporating gentle yoga positions and stretches can improve flexibility, reduce stress, and encourage relaxation.

Tai Chi: This low-impact martial art focuses on slow, deliberate movements that promote balance, coordination, and mindfulness.

Walking: Engaging in regular walks at a reasonable speed can increase cardiovascular health, build muscles, and boost mood without exerting excessive strain on joints.

Swimming or Water Aerobics: Water-based activities provide resistance and support, making them appropriate for persons with joint pain or limited mobility.

Tailoring exercise routines to individual tastes and abilities is critical for fostering adherence and maintaining safety while reaping the advantages of physical activity for autoimmune treatment.

Balancing Movement and Rest

Balancing activity and relaxation are crucial for those with autoimmune disorders to avoid overexertion and manage tiredness. It's crucial to listen to the body's cues and alter activity levels accordingly. Incorporating intervals of rest and recovery between exercise sessions is vital for reducing flare-ups and supporting overall energy levels. Prioritizing adequate sleep and implementing relaxation techniques into everyday routines can help boost recovery and promote general well-being.

Other Lifestyle Factors That Influence Autoimmune Conditions

In addition to exercise and physical activity, several other lifestyle factors can influence autoimmune disorders and general health outcomes:

Nutrition: Following an anti-inflammatory diet rich in nutrient-dense foods helps reduce inflammation, boost immune function, and maximize health outcomes for patients with autoimmune illnesses.

Stress Management: Effective stress-reduction strategies such as mindfulness, meditation, and relaxation can control immunological responses, reduce symptoms, and boost immune resilience.

Sleep Hygiene: Prioritizing adequate and restful sleep is vital for immunological function, inflammatory management, and overall health.

Environmental Factors: Minimizing exposure to environmental toxins, pollutants, and allergens can lessen immune system triggers and support immunological health.

By addressing numerous lifestyle aspects, including exercise, nutrition, stress management, sleep hygiene, and environmental considerations, patients with autoimmune illnesses can adopt a holistic approach to controlling symptoms, enhancing immune function, and boosting overall well-being. Tailoring lifestyle therapies to individual requirements and preferences is crucial to building sustainable habits that support autoimmunity management and long-term health outcomes.

Chapter 7

Case Studies and Success Stories

Case studies and success stories provide essential details into the real-life experiences of individuals who have successfully controlled or conquered autoimmune disorders. These stories illustrate the challenges faced, the solutions adopted, and the successes attained, offering inspiration and practical lessons for others on similar health journeys.

Real-Life Stories of Individuals Who Have Overcome Autoimmune Diseases

Real-life examples of individuals battling autoimmune disorders offer strong narratives of triumph over hardship. These stories generally illustrate personal hardships, moments of breakthroughs, and the transforming impact of lifestyle changes and therapeutic techniques. Through these tales, individuals relate their journeys of diagnosis, problems faced, treatment decisions, and eventually, their routes to recovery or successful disease management.

One such example is that of Elizabeth, a 35-year-old woman diagnosed with rheumatoid arthritis (RA) who struggled with chronic joint pain and tiredness. Sarah's journey began with traditional drugs, but she encountered limited alleviation and undesirable side effects. Determined to recover control of her health, Elizabeth explored alternative therapy, including dietary adjustments and stress-reduction techniques. Over time, Sarah's symptoms improved, and she regained her vitality and quality of life. Her tale stands as a witness to the transforming impact of holistic approaches in controlling autoimmune disorders.

Another encouraging narrative is that of James, a 42-year-old man diagnosed with multiple sclerosis (MS). Facing uncertainties and physical restrictions, James adopted a comprehensive wellness plan that includes regular exercise, mindful eating, and stress management strategies. Through constant dedication and lifestyle improvements, James had a dramatic reduction in MS symptoms, regained mobility, and embraced a fresh sense of empowerment. His tale illustrates the value of tailored health solutions and perseverance in obtaining excellent outcomes.

Lessons Learned and Inspirational Insights

From these real-life examples, several lessons and insights emerge that can aid persons navigating autoimmune diseases:

Empowerment via Education: Many individuals underline the importance of becoming informed about their condition, treatment options, and lifestyle adjustments. Knowledge helps individuals to make educated decisions and actively participate in their health management.

Resilience and Adaptability: Autoimmune journeys typically involve unanticipated hurdles and failures. Resilience and adaptability are crucial skills for negotiating the complexity of chronic illness and finding effective treatments.

Holistic Approaches to Health: Successful outcomes generally arise from holistic approaches that include dietary adjustments, stress reduction measures, exercise, and supportive therapies. Addressing the underlying issues contributing to autoimmune disorders can lead to considerable improvements in symptoms and general well-being.

Community Support: Building a supportive network of healthcare professionals, family, friends, and peers may provide important encouragement, understanding, and assistance throughout the health journey.

Tips for Applying Success Stories to Your Own Health Journey

Applying success stories to one's health journey requires gaining inspiration, learning from others' experiences, and implementing effective techniques. Consider the following methods for utilizing success tales effectively:

Identify Similarities: Identify characteristics of success stories that resonate with your own experiences, challenges, and objectives.

Develop realistic Goals: Break down success stories into concrete stages and develop realistic goals based on individual talents and circumstances.

Seek Guidance: Consult with healthcare professionals or experienced persons for individualized advice and guidance geared to unique health needs.

Stay Persistent: Stay dedicated to implementing lifestyle changes and tactics over time, realizing that results may be gradual and take patience and tenacity.

By utilizing the insights and lessons gleaned from real-life success stories, individuals may empower themselves, create resilience, and make informed choices to support their health journeys toward managing or overcoming autoimmune disorders. Sharing stories and learning from others helps develop a feeling of community, hope, and drive in navigating the intricacies of autoimmune disorders and reaching optimal health results.

Conclusion

In the journey of treating autoimmune diseases and pursuing optimal health, the culmination of experiences, insights, and tactics highlights the necessity of a holistic approach to well-being. Throughout this research, we have delved into the nuances of autoimmune disorders, the importance of nutrition and lifestyle factors, and the inspiring stories of those who have overcome hardship. As we close this discourse, it is important to repeat key topics, offer encouragement, and underline the value of patience, tenacity, and a hopeful approach to overcoming autoimmune health difficulties.

Recap of Key Points and Takeaways

The experience of autoimmune management has revealed numerous essential points and takeaways:

Nutrition Matters: Adopting an anti-inflammatory diet rich in whole foods, prioritizing nutrient-dense options, and avoiding inflammatory triggers can greatly improve autoimmune symptoms and overall well-being.

Lifestyle Factors: Incorporating stress management approaches, regular exercise, decent sleep, and other lifestyle alterations is critical for boosting immune function and controlling autoimmune disorders.

Personalized Approaches: Each individual's health journey is unique. Personalized strategies, informed by medical guidance and self-awareness, play a crucial role in obtaining beneficial outcomes.

Community Support: Building a supportive network of healthcare professionals, family, friends, and peers may provide important encouragement, resources, and solidarity.

Encouragement and Empowerment for Readers

To readers battling autoimmune problems, realize that you are not alone on this road. Your experiences, struggles, and successes build a communal narrative of resilience and optimism. Take courage in knowing that success is possible with informed choices, dedication, and a commitment to holistic health practices. Seek help from reputable sources, advocate for your needs, and embrace the transformative power of lifestyle improvements.

The Importance of Patience and Perseverance

Managing autoimmune disorders needs patience and perseverance. Healing is often nonlinear, having ups and downs along the route. Embrace each step forward, no matter how small, and be compassionate with yourself amid setbacks. Patience offers space for healing, adaptability, and growth. Stay committed to your wellness path, trusting that continuous efforts will deliver positive consequences over time.

A Hopeful Outlook

Maintain a cheerful view on your health journey. Embrace the prospects of improvement, healing, and resilience. Celebrate victories, no matter how gradual, and envisage a future filled with vitality and well-being. Remember that problems are chances for growth, and each day allows making great choices that support your health and happiness.

In conclusion, may this discourse serve as a source of empowerment, inspiration, and practical guidance for persons confronting autoimmune illnesses. Together, let us promote resilience, foster community support, and embrace the transforming potential of holistic health practices. With patience, perseverance, and a hopeful perspective, may each stride forward bring us closer to optimal health and vigorous life.